10 Pounds,
10 Days

by
Chris Miller

ISBN: 978-1-105-67821-9

Table of Contents

Introduction

It started like most things, because some girl had to be impressed.

Her family had purchased a new speed boat. It was mid spring and the cold New England winter was quickly becoming a forgotten memory. To make a long story short they invited me out on the boat, they expected me to go.

Pale, overweight and out of shape was the best way to describe my condition at the time. The thought of being on the boat, out in the ocean, and taking my shirt off to swim or ski made me shiver.

Never mind that I couldn't water ski.

I hated myself then.

For being fat, for letting myself get into this awful state where walking up to my third floor apartment took my breath away. Where I often didn't smile at girls I liked because why would they like a lard ass like me when there are so many other better looking, physically fit guys around.

Her family had just paid for the boat so there was still time before they took possession, maybe a few days, maybe a week if I was lucky. Maybe another week after that before they took it out as a family before bringing friends along. Maybe two weeks total, a window of time in which to drop a few pounds and boost my confidence.

10 pounds in 10 days.

Where the thought came from I couldn't tell you. I didn't even know if it was possible.

But the words kept repeating in my head, becoming my mantra, 10 pounds in 10 days.

10 pounds, 10 days.

Background

To lose a pound of fat 3,500 calories have to be burned or cut out of your diet.

The average person consumes as much as 3,790 calories per day according to the UN Food and Agriculture Organization and without exercising burns approximately 2,000 - 2,700 calories just in the normal course of the days activities.

I am not average.

Between bar tending at a Chinese food restaurant where every meal is fried rice, MSG, chicken wings or beef teryaki, and my lack of a social life which finds me planted firmly behind the TV or computer for the rest of the time I am conscious, I would say that my calorie intake is higher than average. Though 3,790 calories does sound like a lot for an average person to consume my activity level is what I perceive to be well below normal.

And while I am not as overweight as some or as out of shape as others, say the elderly, I still have severe body image issues. Starting this challenge weighing in at 210 pounds, close to my previous all time high of 215, is embarrassing for me. Sure it is a lot lower than others I knew who tried to lose weight, and 40 pounds overweight may not sound like a lot but I hated myself. I needed a change but wasn't desperate enough to lose the weight with some magic weight loss pill.

Losing 10 pounds in 10 days was not going to be done by taking any fat burning supplements, caffeine or diet pills. Those things scare me. There was a time long ago when I took some for a few days. Sure I had more energy only and my urine came out the wrong color and I never really lost much weight.

That shouldn't happen.

Besides which the stories about people dying from taking too much scared me. Just my luck, lose the weight, look great and die the day before I'm supposed to go out on this damn boat.

A pound a day = 3,500 calories.

The question then is to cut 'em or burn 'em.

Cutting the calories could be an option. Fasting is a viable weight loss method and despite what some people believe it can be a very healthy and rewarding experience when done properly. When I was younger I often fasted for a couple days at a time for religious reasons. You would not believe the amount of energy you have after the second day of fasting when your body is freed from digesting until you experience it first hand.

But fasting for the whole ten days?

Even considering a juice fast, where you are allowed to drink juice in addition to water to help you through made me question whether or not the will power would be there. Fasting seems to amplify not just the smell of food but turned every fast food commercial into pornography.

Its not like the weight would be gained back once the fast was over. That's one of the greatest misconceptions about fasting. Sure you do gain some weight back, but not all of it. People think that it is water weight that you lose, but during a proper fast you consume far more water than the average person.

And water weight is heavy.

But fasting to lose the ten pounds in ten days wasn't for me.

Burning the 3,500 calories seemed like a better option. Sitting behind a TV or in front of the computer for marathon length stretches of time hadn't done anything for my state of physical well being.

I was a blob, soft like pudding.

The thought of physical fitness regimes that would be required made me cringe. Like everyone else I had joined a gym years ago to try and shed some pounds. That lasted maybe three weeks, with a few scattered visits before I gave up and canceled my membership.

It wasn't that the gym didn't work or that I didn't feel or look better, I did. Going to the gym simply wasn't my thing. Besides which I was usually too hung over to go early in the morning with my gym partner.

And a partner can be motivation.

Being a bartender I tend to work later, into the AM, and drink even later. Maybe if I cut out drinking I could seriously cut out a bunch of calories. After all vodka alone is 75 or so calories a fluid ounce, of which I will consume at least ten ounces chased with Coca Cola, adding another 700 or so calories to the mix.

We're talking 1,400 to 1,500 calories per day from drinking alone.

Burning all of the calories didn't seem like the right way to go either. It looked like I was going to have to do a combination of the two if I was going to lose 10 pounds in ten days.

The first order of business would be reducing my calorie intake and eating healthier.

I wasn't going to put down any structured meal plan or count calories or carb's or anything like that. I know from experience that I'll start doing that and cheat and give up within a few days. Most likely calling the diet plan a bunch of crap anyway.

I would just consciously try to eat less, drink less and, hardest part, cut out the candy, chocolate and ice cream for a while.

Working at the Chinese food restaurant much of the food is fried and most of the dishes that are cooked in the wok contain sugar and worse, MSG.

It doesn't help that the food is free.

You probably already know that MSG, mono sodium glutamate, is a flavor enhancer used in more foods than the average person would believe possible. In fact it is one of the most widely used food additives in the world. Besides giving some people headaches research has shown that it may interfere with appetite regulation. People who consume large amounts of it tend to be heavier than others consuming the same amount of calories.

No more fried foods for lunch or dinner while working, or at home for that matter.

Like a lot of people I barely ever cook a meal at home. It is just infinitely easier to go out for a meal than to have to do the grocery shopping and prep work that goes into making a meal. So healthier options are somewhat limited, but not impossible.

I also tend to drink a lot of soda. Since diet sodas contain aspartame as a way to reduce calories, that is not an option when trying to lose weight. At least for me. There is quite a little aspartame controversy going on about its health effects, and some believe, that like MSG, it alters your appetite control or changes the bodies ability to utilize the food it does consume.

So instead of diet soda I would just try to limit the intake of regular soda, hopefully below my current 2 liters a day.

Back the the burn 'em part of the calorie count.

Exercise is not one of my favorite things. I have weights and a curling bar in my bedroom. They have been there since I moved. In fact they have been untouched in the last three apartments I have lived in. They don't get used because even though I say I'm going to get back in shape I just never do it.

Besides which weight lifting doesn't burn enough calories for my 10 day challenge. Sure it may improve my physical appearance and self confidence but its not for me.

Swimming burns roughly 700 or more calories per hour but it also requires access to a pool, which without a gym or YMCA membership is not an option.

Running is also an option, I used to be in track as a freshman and sophomore in high school. So what if that was 20 years ago. Then I remember running a few years ago when I was in one of those, "It's time to get back in shape" type moods.

I remember the concrete sidewalk slamming under my feet, the burning pain coursing through my muscles as I gasped for breath, spitting thick saliva and feeling like I wanted to die.

Despite burning 700 or so calories calories per hour, running wasn't my cup of tea either.

Walking was more pleasant and there was the paved, off road Blackstone River Bikeway nearby that would be perfect for it, only walking burns 350 calories per hour at a fast pace, and only 200 calories per hour at a slower pace. I would have to do a hell of a lot of walking everyday to get anywhere near my 10 pounds in 10 days goal even if I did significantly cut my calorie intake.

Cycling on the other hand burns between 500 and 900 calories per hour depending on your pace. That still adds up to hell of a lot of time on the bike just to burn enough calories. Even if I manage to bike early so that I benefit from the increased metabolism throughout the rest of the day it still means four hours to get anywhere near the 3,500 calories I need to burn.

There was a study I had read that said if you managed to do a cardio workout early in the day it would actually boost your metabolism throughout the entire day. Sort of like a delayed and extra benefit.

They call it "Afterburn".

Not only does it increase your metabolism throughout the day but getting that exercise out of the way is a tremendous load off of your mind. I wouldn't have to worry about doing it after work knowing I would probably just put it off for another day because all I wanted to do was relax.

Getting some cardio exercise in early on the bike had another advantage, with low levels of blood sugar from not eating all night it is much easier to burn fat. One study suggested that you burn up to three times as much fat when doing cardio with low morning blood sugar levels when you do a minimum of 30 minutes.

And with the completed 10 mile portion of the Blackstone River Bikeway almost next door to my house it would be hard to think of an excuse not to ride. The hard part would be getting in the bike ride early in the day.

When I was a kid I used to like biking everywhere. Of course that was before I had a car.

Being in New England, cycling is something can only be done during the summer months unless you are one of those die hard cyclists that has to be out on the road in all conditions.

I haven't been on a bike in five years. Back then I thought of biking to work to cut down on gas costs, get a little exercise and help save the environment. That's when I found out that I suffered from a terrible curse known simply as flat-tire-itis. It is a condition that causes even new inner tubes to magnetically attract sharp objects and go flat.

For those genetically predisposed to this horrendous disease the treatment, frequent replacement of inner tubes can be a costly affair.

Between constantly replacing inner tubes and being hit by a car that was not paying attention, leaving me gasping for breath in the middle of a street, my brief stint as a bicycle commuter came to a end.

But the bike path was right there, and cycling burned so many calories.

Could I do it?

Besides which the Blackstone River Bikeway was a paved off road bike path, I didn't have to worry about someone in a car not paying attention running me off the road or worse, smearing me across the asphalt.

I pulled my old bike out of storage, the tires looked like they were still inflated because they had solid core inner tubes, they're like giant rubber O rings that go inside your tire, no air, no flats. Curse be damned. I hit the bike path, even in the lower gears I could feel how out of shape I was. Breathing deep gulps of air didn't seem to help. I was winded and I wasn't even a half mile down the path. Fighting every headwind, wondering if I was really this far out of shape.

Home never felt better.

After a cool down outside my apartment I realized that I would now have to carry the bike up three flights of stairs. I had never realized how heavy and awkward the bike was and the thought of doing that everyday, bringing it up and down the stairs just to ride had me thinking second thoughts.

There is no way that is going to happen everyday.

Lets be realistic.

Upstairs it was obvious that the bike needed to be cleaned and oiled from sitting in storage for so long. Maybe I wasn't as out of shape as seemed obvious, maybe the bike just reluctantly dragged itself along for the ride. It was apparent that this bike needed a tune up, but even then would it fit the bill? It was an older model, heavy as hell and well, ugly.

"Am I going to do it, lose 10 pounds in 10 days, or am I going to wimp out?" My brain asked.

Or more accurately, accused.

The thought of the excuses I would have to make to get out of going out on the boat, of not being able to be comfortable around the girl after that made me go to the bike shop and buy a new bike.

Granted it was a bottom of the line mountain bike for less than $150, but at least it wasn't a Wal-mart bike. Spending too much on a bike and unnecessary accessories that may end up as a clothes rack was not something that that I wanted to do.

I still didn't want to admit that this was an experiment. Maybe it was a phase, there had been others, the pickles instead of chips diet, the healthy milkshake for breakfast diet... I could go on but the list gets depressing when I think about all the attempts that failed.

The frame of the bike was a little too small for me at 16" but I had the idea of storing the bike in my car instead of carrying up and down three flights of stairs every time I wanted to go for a ride to burn some calories. Besides which this bike was 15 pounds lighter than the old bike. (the scale in my bathroom is getting a lot of use this week.) The bike fits nice in the back of my station wagon and as I pulled into my parking spot I was still wondering if I could do this.

No time like the present.

I looked at myself in the rear view mirror. Seriously?

Why not?

And there was no reason why I couldn't go for a ride right now.

The bike was out of the car and on the bike path before I could second guess myself. I rode farther and felt better than I had on my old bike. The new black and shiny bike seemed to glide across the pavement, down the bike lane made for... well, bikes.

I wondered at the feel of the wind in my face, the way the least amount of physical exertion seemed to speed me along further down the path, closer to my goal. I would be seeing her, there on the boat, like I imagined, like I worried about.

Only now everything was better.

Everything was going to be all right if I kept riding.

And I actually had fun.

Sure I was still a little winded, my heart rate was up and I could feel a little burn in my legs, but I didn't push myself. I had to stay positive.

"You're not fat, just out of shape... and overweight."

This might actually work.

It starts tomorrow. Tonight at work I eat and drink like normal and tomorrow the 10 pounds in 10 days challenge begins.

Day 1

Awake, laying in my bed listening to the guys across the street playing soccer and wondering if it was really possible to lose 10 pounds in 10 days. Was I crazy? Why was I doing this to myself? The thought of her forced me out of the bed and outside.

The thought of her on that damn boat.

The sound of the water gently slapping against the side of the boat as it rocked ever so slightly, she was laying out on a towel.

In a bikini.

Her skin exposed to the sun.

And my fat ass laying in bed.

The bike came out of the car easily and seemed lighter than the day before when I bought it. It's just a piece of lightweight aluminum, a piece of metal. A tool.

In the cool morning before sunrise I considered a digital meter for tracking time and distance, maybe they had one that kept track of calories burned. It wasn't long before my heart rate was up and I was sweating from the exertion of peddling the bike. I was up earlier than usual and totally enjoying myself.

The "hills" on the Blackstone River Bikeway aren't really hills. More like elongated humps. But the wind, the damn wind killed me.

"I could do this," I kept repeating, "I can do this. Just keep peddling."

My confidence level seemed a little higher than it had been in weeks. This was possible, it was going to happen. It was happening.

Without having to worry about cars and auto traffic riding was fun. If it wasn't for the labored breathing I would have felt like a kid again.

Right now the Blackstone River Bikeway is 10 miles of off road paved bike path going from The Cumberland/Central falls line through Lincoln and up into Woonsocket. Eventually it will be 48 miles long and go all the way north into Worcester, MA and south into Providence, RI. The section that I ride follows the old Providence and Worcester Railroad line and the long defunct Blackstone Canal which runs along side the river.

It is the local section of the East Coast Greenway, a 2,900 mile trail system that connects Maine to Florida and hopes to be the handicapped accessible version of the popular Appalachian Trail. The fact that this little path is just one part of a plan to create an off road route that links the major cities of the east coast blows my mind.

Imagine being able to ride the entire way, as far south as Key West on one bicycle route?

Long distance touring bicyclists can burn as much as 6,000 calories or more per day. How much weight would you lose then? How much would you be able to eat every day and not ever show the slightest weight gain? Would the hard part be controlling your appetite, or do you just pig out at any buffet you can find?

I smiled and hoped that I would get the chance to find out. Maybe ride the whole thing after this summer is over, after I'm in shape and feeling better about myself.

Isn't that what they say? Set a big goal.

I will ride a long distance bike trip when this is said and done.

If I "like" cycling that is.

"Why do you always have to qualify everything?" My brain immediately asked.

I rode on in silence for a little while with no response.

"Just focus on losing the 10 pounds in 10 days," I had to remind myself, "this is only Day 1."

An unexpected benefit to the ride was that it cleared my head out of all the noise from work and life. I had no cell phone with me so there was no way anyone could interrupt. I was free to let my thoughts wander, and they did with startling clarity.

My mind jumped back to a fact I had heard about coconut oil, that it was supposed to help you lose weight. Over a year ago I had thought the idea was so simple that it couldn't have worked, it was absurd. But it was such a simple idea, take a tablespoon full of virgin coconut oil in the morning and one in the afternoon that I eventually thought why not give it a try.

A tablespoon twice a day.

That's it.

So I bought a jar of coconut oil, the problem was that when it is cold out the coconut oil solidifies. So I had to gently warm it up every time I wanted to take a spoonful off the top. I did this for a few days in the morning, skipping the afternoon spoonful because I was out working or running some errand.

After five days my pants were literally sliding off me. My size 34 jeans at the time seemed a little loose, and when I went to the store found that I could now fit into a size 32. In less than a week the coconut oil had made a vast difference in my appearance.

I don't know how it worked, but it did.

That little problem of having to heat the coconut oil up every time soon wore me out and I stopped taking spoonfuls of it every morning. At first I would continue to take it when I remembered, then the jar got pushed to the back of the cabinet and forgotten. Since I had already reaped the benefits it was quickly forgotten.

"But what if it came in capsule form?", my mind wondered as I pedaled away a few more calories. If I could get some of those and take them with my vitamins every morning it would infinitely easier than the heating thing and I might even stick with it.

I resolved to get some and include it in the 10 day challenge.

After riding for a while I couldn't concentrate as much, it felt like I was hunched over awkwardly. I stopped briefly on the path to look at my seat, it was angled ever so slightly forward which is unnoticeable on shorter rides but now that I was trying to ride longer and burn more calories the slight angle was painfully obvious.

The benefits of buying your bike from a good bike dealer being that they will fit your body to the proper sized bike. Lets face it, we all have different body types, some have long arms and legs, others shorter legs and longer torso's.

Most of the pain of starting to ride can be avoided by proper sizing of the bike for a better overall riding position.

Seat height is another important consideration. Too low and you will over strain your knees.

To find the right height sit on the bike with your feet on the peddles. The lower leg pushed all the way to the bottom of the pedal rotation should still be bent at the knee by 25 to 30 degrees max.

No more, no less.

The seat should also be level.

Handle bars should be even with or slightly lower than the level of your seat. No more than an inch or two.

I cringe when I see people with their seats far below their handle bars, not only is it straining their knees but they aren't even really getting the workout that they think they are.

You should be loose and relaxed with your elbows slightly bent.

Higher handlebars can reduce strain on the lower back if you are serious about putting in some time burning calories on the bike and your body hasn't quite adjusted to the physical exercise.

After the ride I hit the shower and weighed myself, 208. I couldn't believe it. Had yesterdays little ride burned a few calories? I certainly hadn't altered anything I ate, we had baked salt wings last night for dinner. Kind of like the regular fried wings but these are battered, fried, then tossed in a wok with salt, scallions and jalapenos. Dessert was a couple dozen Hershey Caramel Kisses and a chocolate Frosty from Wendy's.

Not exactly diet food.

Just thinking about all the food I had last night was making me hungry. Indeed I seemed to be a little more hungry than usual. I put it of my mind and tried to get some stuff done on the computer before I had to run out and do some errands.

Feeling like I had more energy than usual I left the computer and went out. Before I knew it I was sitting at the bar. Out of habit I had sat myself in one of my favorite places to read, a chain restaurant that makes great long island iced teas. I had considered drinking something else since I was supposed to be losing 10 pounds over the next 10 days but the bartender already had it made, she saw me coming and I never order anything else.

Oh well right, what's a few calories. But I was also still much more hungry than usual. Nothing on the menu seemed like enough. Vowing to "really" start the challenge tomorrow I ordered a 10 ounce sirloin steak with loaded mashed potatoes, extra butter and a side of onion rings.

If I was going to screw with the challenge then I was really going to do it.

It wasn't to long after that where I fell back into my old ways, sitting on my fat ass watching movies and having a few drinks. Except I drank far more than a few and watched several movies.

Not really an active lifestyle.

Day 1:

7 Miles

45 Minutes

Day 2

"This cant be right", I thought to myself when I weighed in the morning of Day 2.

206 pounds?

I didn't cut back on eating like I wanted, having the steak, loaded mashed potatoes, onion rings and a long island iced tea at lunch. And after that I had consumed almost half of a 750 ml bottle of vodka and a 2 liter bottle of coke.

The vodka and soda alone that were consumed last night accounted for almost 1,700 calories.

Putting the 10 day challenge off had made me feel like a fraud, like I was the same old person who had failed to keep up with all those diets, all those times before.

206 pounds.

Maybe the bike thing would work.

Take my vitamins with water instead of the usual milk. Not because I'm being good about calories but because I drank the last of the milk last night when I finished off a half gallon of tin roof sundae ice cream.

Coconut pills, multi vitamin.

Downstairs I get the bike out of the car, so much easier than trying to carry it up and down the three flights of stairs through the cramped hallway. It's such a tight in fit in the hall that I had to give away my luxurious queen size mattress when I moved in because it simply wouldn't fit around the corners of the hallway. I settled for a single size mattress.

Its not like I'd be having any sleep overs with my lack of self confidence.

Today I was prepared.

I brought down the vice grips and straightened out the seat to keep me more level and to make the ride more comfortable.

That today was different was apparent as soon as I sat on the bike.

My ass hurt.

Sitting on the seat was uncomfortable but bearable. I still had to ride, had to see this thing through. Maybe it would just take me a few days to get my rear end used to riding again.

Then when I started to peddle I felt the burn in my leg muscles that I didn't feel before. I had intended on riding past Martin Street Bridge where I had eventually turned around the day before, wanted to see what I could really do, but with the burn in my legs I started to second guess myself.

I knew that somewhere up ahead there was a historic landmark called Kelley House, I wasn't sure how much farther it was but it would make a decent landmark, if I could make it. I cut those thoughts off right away before they got out of hand.

"You said you're riding farther today and that's what you're going to do."

End of discussion.

No excuses.

The morning was fantastic. The sun was out and I hadn't been awake at 8am in at least a few months. There was no reason for me to be up that early, especially after drinking all night long. But sitting in bed wasn't an option, there were calories to be burned.

There was a chill when I started riding but between the rising sun and the exercise from the bike I wasn't worried. A little over a mile into the bike path the Department of Environmental Management had a truck and a couple of saw horses blocking the path.

I couldn't believe it, I know there had been some damage to the path from the recent flooding, between the snow melt and a recent rain storm that dropped 3 to 5 inches of rain over night the Blackstone River was well above flood levels. The images of local flooding had been all over the news with over 500 cars being submerged in Warwick alone.

There was no choice but to turn around and circle around on streets until I got to another access point for the bike path. Worse than the cars, the street route would take me over a hill far steeper than any I would encounter on the bike path. A hill that was probably nothing to any regular cyclist, this thing was going to be a challenge for my newly forming leg muscles.

"I never met a hill I couldn't walk up."

I don't know who said it or where I heard it but I thought worse comes to worse I could get off and walk the bike. Halfway up the hill I had to shift down for the third time. Watching every pebble and discarded empty soda bottle slowly pass by I considered getting off of the bike.

Then I down shifted again and in the most authoritative voice I could muster said to myself, "Just peddle stupid."

The alternate route wasn't as far as I had thought it was going to be and soon the path was beneath the bikes tires again. Kelly house here we come. Before I knew it I was at the Martin Street Bridge where I turned around and headed back the day before.

Today I was going farther.

Then my heart sank when I saw the orange cones and florescent orange tape seemingly blocking the bike path. Was the damage going to prevent me from going further now that I had decided to push on? Was I doomed never to lose this weight?

A closer look at the caution signs as I approached made it clear that though some of the path had been washed away there was still a single lane open. Only the Kelly House wasn't that much farther past the bridge.

Turning around now seemed stupid.

As I cross the bridge at Kelly House I notice that the Blackstone river is a few shades light yellow than it is down river, looking less like dirty urine but still obviously polluted.

At this point in the ride I realize two things, if I am going to be on the bike for over an hour I should remember to bring a water bottle. The cheap bike I bought was bare bones and didn't even come with a mounted water bottle or cage.

And number two, I really should have had at least brought a light snack with me even though I was trying to burn more calories with the low blood sugar exercise. The retired stripper with hand weights out for a lonely morning walk made my empty stomach do flip flops from the cloud of perfume that surrounded her like a toxic gas.

At least she was on the right side of the path.

Trail etiquette is not a high priority it seems. Despite signs everywhere telling walkers to stay to the left to face oncoming bicycles they continue to walk on the right as if they were in a car. They don't see you coming and they don't pay enough attention to their kids running around blocking the path.

I was beginning to realize that just because the path was off road didn't mean it was free of hassles, and was thinking about turning around when I came to the point where the bike path has a couple of right angles in it to cross the railroad tracks. Memorable, and as good a point as any to call it a day, until I look ahead and see the hill.

"You're going to turn around because you don't want to ride up the hill", my brain whispers.

Dammit.

Down shifting a few gears I climb the hill, slowly, standing to get some extra power while pain shoots through what I imagine are my sensitive reproductive organs and flabby white ass. Over the hill and across another bridge I decide to keep going as far as the dam which I know is somewhere up ahead.

Standing next to the still swollen river pouring over the dam the water looks even less like piss than it did just a mile or two earlier. How far up would a person have to go so that the water was no longer yellow as it poured over rocks and dams?

Did the bike path go that far?

The dam was just across the bridge on the other side of the hill. I turned around and headed back attempting to ride while standing up a few more times. Not because I was trying to get the hang of it but because my ass and crotch hurt so much I had to stand to try and relieve some of the pain.

Then back at the house after the ride the strangest thing happened. My lower stomach area around my belly button became extremely itchy all the way to the sides of my body.

It was a painful burning itch.

I splashed my stomach down with water and tried to itch away some of the feeling but the whole area turned red, bright, scary red. After several long agonizing minutes the itched faded but my skin was raised in small bumps. The panic subsided. I don't know what caused it, was it my stomach rubbing against itself while sweating and bent over for a long period of time, was it the extreme amount of calories I'd just burned?

That just seemed silly.

Since I was trying to keep it calorie light today I held myself to a quart of 1% milk and a couple of tablespoons full of raw honey for breakfast. You might find that a little odd since honey is basically just sugar to most people. But honey not only cuts my cravings for chocolate but it also metabolizes differently than refined sugars.

That's what I'd read anyway, so I justified it as a way curb my insatiable love for chocolate.

As far as the butt pain, Gel bike seat covers slide around a lot. That's what the owner of the bike store was telling me.

"On long distance rides they also cut off blood to places where you are supposed to have blood go." She added.

The other option was padded bike shorts. Nothing like a giant pad in your underwear to make you feel special. She suggests I buy a pair with flat stitching to prevent chafing, "Maybe In the $80 range." she says looking through the rack explaining that chafing is "bad".

"That's a little more than I was expecting." I said looking at the prices for myself.

She cant find any under $99, luckily I spot a pair with regular stitching for $50. I hesitated before buying them, did I really need them or should I just tough it out for another few rides until my ass gets used to riding the bike?

I threw them on the counter and asked about bike computers for tracking speed and mileage. She hands me a low cost one and I ask about calorie counting as a function.

"This other model here is a little more expensive but has a calorie counter, I'm not too sure how accurate it is though." she adds watching me check the price tag.

"Doesn't really matter," I say putting the more expensive model back down on the display case, "its not that that important." I say paying for the shorts and meter with no calorie counter because I don't want to admit that I am a fat ass cycling to lose weight.

Together the shorts and computer set me back slightly more than half the cost of the entire bike.

This is getting to be an expensive challenge.

Back at home I try the bike shorts on, if you have never worn a pair of padded bicycle shorts imagine a smooth fluffy taco shell trying to press its way out of your ass crack. Yes, just like that. It's like having a giant maxi pad for your butt sewn to the inside of your underwear.

All of a sudden I wasn't so sure the padded shorts were such a good idea.

The bike computer takes longer to attach than I anticipated, and while trying to set it my landlord comes over and wants to talk screwing me up and forcing me to have to reprogram it all over again. I can't remember what he said, something about rent or an alien invasion, I don't know, I was too distracted by the taco trying to escape from my ass.

At least once I was on the bike it was hard to notice the pad at all, if it wasn't for the lack of pain I wouldn't have known it was there. I had just finished lunch, a 6 inch turkey sub from Subway, extra lettuce, light mayo, vinegar, and I figured I would take the bike out for a test run with the new shorts.

Besides which two rides in one day couldn't hurt the calorie burn.

The bike path is very different at 5:30 pm compared to the earlier rides I had been doing. First off there are a hell of a lot more people. People who had just returned home from work, families with their kids now home from school. And with more people there are more who don't know what side of the path to walk on. Worse than that a group of people will block the way and only reluctantly move. Two people walking will walk next to each other talking and take up the whole path. The worst by far for me was the 20 something couple riding bikes side by side who refused to go single file when other oncoming bikes would pass.

Unbelievable.

Then I remember that Massachusetts and Rhode Island have the worst drivers in the country and realize that this extends to riding bikes and even to walking.

Even with all the extra people and being tired from the ride earlier I managed to make it out to the Martin Street bridge and back in only 33 minutes compared to the 45 minutes it took me on Day 1. My chest swelling with pride, well maybe not swelling, I was having a hard time inhaling. It wasn't a shortness of breath, just a tightness in my chest.

To inhale hurt. As if my lung capacity diminished due to an itchy sort of hurting feeling deep down in the back of my throat. Shallow breaths hurt less but didn't seem to supply the amount of oxygen my body needed.

This is new.

The fact that my body needed oxygen. I'd never had to think about breathing before, except the rare head cold where you are so stuffed up it is impossible to breathe through your nose. It's like you are suffocating, or how I imagine it is to have an asthma attack.

It wasn't scary really, more like a sign of progress. A painful sign of progress.

After doing so good earlier in the day calorie wise I still managed to end the night bad. They were spicy garlic BBQ chicken wings. My friend had made them and she wanted me to eat a bunch.

"One." I said, but she had cooked them to split with me.

I ended up eating more than a few.

And we had drinks. Not as much as I had the night of Day 1 but enough that its a significant amount of calories that could have been avoided.

Why am I weakening around food and drinks? Am I not taking this challenge seriously?

Food and drinks. Drinks and food.

And yet there is that angry little part of me that doesn't want to do the challenge. The part that wants to take it easy and be lazy and eat and drink all the time, to sit on the couch and watch movies. The little voice says, "Where is the crime in that?"

"Why does other peoples judgment about my weight make me hate myself and not them? They after all are judging me. Why should I suffer to make them happy."

That little, quiet, nagging voice wants me to give up, to surrender before this thing has even begun. It keeps reminding me that 3,500 calories a day is a big chunk to make disappear, and I haven't been biking enough, I'm not in shape enough and I have been drinking too much.

Back at home, alone, with no air conditioning the apartment is sweltering. The window is open with the barest hint of a breeze lightly brushing the screen. Laughing I realize that the new bike computer has a temperature gauge on it. If I had the bike upstairs I would know how hot it was in my room making me sweat.

But carrying the bike upstairs is too much work.

All my plans on cutting back on the calorie intake are in the toilet, being flushed by an overweight steak house chef, laughing maniacally as he watches me eat more, and more, and more...

At least the drinks are on the house.

Day 2:

First Ride

12.6 Miles

1 Hour 30 Minutes

Second Ride

7 Miles

33 Minutes

Day 3

Friends don't let friends eat BBQ when they are trying to lose weight.

Despite being down another pound from the day before the guilt of eating so much the night before weighed heavily on my mind.

As punishment for last nights binge I have decided to do the unthinkable.

To push past any semblance of a learning curve and push myself into oblivion. I want my muscles to burn. I want to feel the pain.

Pain is weakness leaving the body.

The now dry padded cycling shorts were still propped up on the 2 liter soda bottle where I placed them to air out after washing them last night. I knew before leaving that I was going to push myself today but I wasn't sure how much.

I stole the water bottle cage off of my old bike and put it on the new one. A 1 liter Poland Spring water bottle fit perfectly, and water would be a requirement today.

Breakfast was simple, vitamins, coconut oil, and a glass of 1% milk. At least the gallon is still more than halfway full. Usually if a gallon of milk lasts more than two days it means that I have been working too much.

Cruising along the bike path I wondered how hard I should push myself. My legs don't burn like they did yesterday even though they do feel different. The pace is faster than usual but I'm feeling optimistic, dare I think about doing the whole bike path?

Just as I'm thinking, "Yeah lets try for the whole thing", the path is blocked by barriers and Environmental Management people doing work on the Martin Street Bridge.

More damage, more repairs.

So I take the path up to street level and start to bike parallel to the path on the street and re-enter the path not much further up by Kelly House.

Here we go, to the end. No matter what.

I couldn't have picked a better day to push myself, it was clear, warm but not hot, and there weren't that many people out on the bike path. The railroad still runs on the tracks that run parallel with much of the bike path and I raced along next to the three orange and brown engines pulling at least fifty tankers full of ethanol.

OK, I cheated, I looked up the hazard codes when I got home from the ride.

I joined the cluster of people at the railroad crossing waiting for it to go by so they could continue their walk or ride.

Everyone seemed like they were in a good mood.

I knew I was nearing the end when I passed the water treatment plant I had seen from the road when a friend and I scouted the route from their car. "Not much further I thought", then I realized that even when I reach the end it will still only be halfway through the ride.

At the end of the finished section of the bike path in Woonsocket is the River's Edge Recreational Complex. With soccer fields and a couple of golf greens thrown in for fun the sign by the bike path said they had vending machines and bathrooms. Instantly I had a craving for a Snickers bar. Then I realized that I didn't have any money, not even a credit card since I left my wallet at home.

At first I thought the path might continue further since the mile marker posts were marked for 14 miles and yet I had only done 11 miles. But there it was, a stone floored circle at the end of the path.

I did two loops around it and headed back.

Coming back there was a head wind that slowed me down and made me work harder just to maintain a decent speed. I just wanted the ride to be over. I was tired and losing focus, at times it was like I forgot that I was on a bike at all. I would stop pedaling, my mind completely blank and just drift.

Then the bike would slow down so much I would snap out of it and start peddling again.

My crotch really hurt too.

The padded shorts were working but it felt like the seat was angled up into me. Stopping at Manville Dam for a much needed stretch, the seat looked level, maybe I need to angle it down again just a little to take some of the pressure off.

It felt like someone had my urethra in a pair of vice grips. I don't think I could have pee'd if I'd wanted to.

The water at Manville Dam was worse than the water downstream. It still had that yellow tint but here it was more of a deep brown color. And it smelled. The spray from the dam insured that scent got around. I stretched and watched a couple of tires and a propane tank playing at the base of the falls, swimming into the falls to be forced underwater only to reappear a minute later and do it all over again.

Towards the end of the ride I was trying to stand to relieve some of the pressure of the seat pressing into me when I noticed that my foot was shaking on the pedal. My legs were feeling the burn as well and I wondered what it would be like when I got off the bike.

Would I even be able to stand?

Back at home my legs were quivering and it seemed like I might collapse when I tried walking. My hands were shaking when I took the car keys out of my pocket, everything felt like rubber and it was clear that I did not have full control of my limbs.

Looking at the bike computer I realized that not only did I do the whole bike path, I kept a 12mph average and finished the almost 22 miles in only an hour and 48 minutes.

That's almost twice the distance as yesterdays first ride and only 18 minutes longer.

Getting the bike into the back of the car was a chore and I felt like a zombie getting up to my apartment, leaning against the wall for support as I made my way upstairs. My head went under the cold water in the kitchen sink as I continued to shake and tremble.

But damn, I did it, rode the whole bike path from end to end.

Day 3:

22 Miles

1 Hour 48 Minutes

Day 4

The scale in the bathroom said 204 pounds.

I had lost 6 pounds already.

This was amazing, more than I could have hoped for, and with the day off of work I decided to try a new bike path, still part of the East Coast Greenway but a different stretch further south. It was the Washington Secondary Bike Path which is a rail trail that runs along the old Providence, Hartford, & Fishkill Railroad that was made up of several smaller bike paths connected together passing through Cranston, Warwick, West Warwick and Coventry.

What I liked was that they have all been linked together into a single, mostly paved, off road path.

The problem was that it was supposed to rain all day, maybe slowing down at 8pm according to the Weather Channel. But I couldn't skip a day, I had to keep the momentum going, the results were too impressive.

So I went to work on the computer, looking for directions to the trail and keeping an eye on the rain. Then, magically it seemed to stop. From inside the apartment, peering out the window I wasn't sure if it was the end of the rain or only a temporary reprieve.

Who cares. I shut down the computer and bounded down the stairs clutching the handwritten directions, the only ones I could find online, and headed towards my car.

Outside though it had started sprinkling again.

"I'm going to get wet not matter what", I thought and decided to go anyway.

As soon as my car pulled on the highway the downpour started. Thick sheets of rain that made driving the speed limit impossible and made me wonder if I was going to get to try out the new path.

Weather wasn't something I'd thought to take into account when I considered losing weight.

The other problem, besides the rain, was that the only directions I could find online were to a place in Warwick that ended up being almost in the middle of the bike path. There were no signs posted at the parking area so it was a guess as to which way to go first. At the time I didn't know I was in the dead center of the bike path, I thought the longer way was to the north, back towards Cranston and turned my bike in that direction.

The rain had stopped soon after I arrived. Sure there were puddles everywhere and I was still going to get wet because I hadn't invested in fenders but at least I was going to ride.

Headed north on the trail I looked forward to what appeared to be a miles long gradual incline. Not even a half a mile into the ride my thighs were burning and I wast sure how much of the ride I was going to be able to complete.

At least coming back would be all downhill.

The rain seemed to have kept most people away and for a while it was if I had the entire bike path all to myself. Sure there was a girl coming home from school, a guy coming back from the supermarket so engrossed in his phone that he may not have even seen me go by and a few other stragglers walking their dogs, holding umbrellas to protect them from the light drizzle that had started up again.

There was nothing to aggravate me besides the cross walk lights taking far too long to change. I was eager to keep moving, everything was so beautiful and I was in such a good mood.

The ride back I started to feel better, there was no burning pain in my thighs anymore and my seat adjustment seemed to be taking some of the pressure off of my butt. Granted my arms were taking up some of that pressure because I could feel it in my shoulders and triceps, but I could live with that.

As I reached my car it was still fairly clear out and I felt good, it was only another 4 miles to the West Warwick end of the path so I passed my car and kept going. No sooner than I had decided to see the other end of the bike path than the clouds opened up and released a heavy rain.

I had to laugh, because before I could even consider turning around my brain whispered "You better not even think about turning around", so I kept on, through the cold and well... wet rain.

Of course it was wet, it is water.

Duh.

According to the bike computer it was 51 degrees out and I was soaking wet. The wind gusts added a nice little chill.

Heading south from that point is mostly uphill. Because it was an old rail line it can only be so steep, but you have to work going in that direction. It was as if I had chosen the lowest elevation point in the entire trail to park my car.

At the end of the finished portion of the bike path, after the climb, there was another section extending the path that was under construction. Eventually this will be the longest, continuously paved, off road bike path in Rhode Island.

For now I just made a mental note that if I was doing this ride again from end to end starting from the Garfield Street parking lot in Cranston would be the best bet. That way the long climb to West Warwick is in the middle of the trip and not the end.

After the ride there was no trembling in my legs, though I did notice some tingling in my hands from having to take on some extra weight because of the slightly tilted forward bike seat.

I wiped down the chain and as much of the bike as possible with napkins from my glove compartment and when I took off my sweatshirt it weighed half as much as the bike. Wringing out as much water as I could from the sweatshirt I turned on the heat and headed home.

Only it was rush hour and the traffic was stop and go. My thigh started to burn from the constant switching between gas and braking. When I rubbed it I realized that my whole thigh hurt to the touch.

That and my hands were beyond numb and tingling on the steering wheel.

When I finally got home my first attempt at lifting my leg out of the car didn't work.

I had to use my tingling hands to help lift it out and set it on the ground. Reluctantly the right leg followed. One step at a time I made it up to my apartment in an agonizing slow march. Pulling my wet jeans and socks off was a monumental task. My hands were pins and needles, painful to the touch with an eerie kind of numbness that made them feel partially paralyzed.

The numbness in my hands lasted for about two hours after the ride, so much for the seat adjustment.

And I did better calorie wise that day than on any other day. You'd think that after that much pain and suffering that I would deserve something good, a decent treat to acknowledge the fact that I had done a good job. But quite the opposite, I saw no reason to ruin what had been a decent amount of calories burned.

Let the pain be its own reward.

Day 4:
21.18 Miles
1 Hour 43 Minutes

Day 5

204 pounds?

After being so good calorie wise the day before and getting in almost two hours on the bike I had expected some kind of drop. I couldn't help but wonder if the now obvious extra leg muscles I could feel were skewing the weigh in.

Muscle weighs more than fat. If I was adding muscle I was adding weight.

I can't give up now, I'm halfway through, day wise and weight wise.

I did have to work later so any riding today would have to be a shorter trip. Having enjoyed the Washington Secondary Bike Path the day before I thought I would try another new bike path before I got bored with the one right outside my door. The O'Neil Bike Path from Kingston station was a bit shorter at only 7 miles long but I wanted to give my body a little rest from the abuse it had suffered through the day before.

There wasn't much information about the bike path online, directions seemed simple enough, but with it being so far away and such a short trail I knew this would probably be the first and last time I saw it.

Being a Saturday there were tons of people out crowding the bike path. It seemed to be a constant climb in one direction until the end where the as yet unfinished path continued on streets. After a little exploring I lost where the trail should go and decided to head back.

Only it seemed to be uphill in this direction as well.

Why does the bike path always look like it is uphill?

It felt like I couldn't catch a break.

Back at the car in about an hour I wanted to turn around and do it again. Only I had to get to work, didn't want to end up stuck in rush hour traffic again.

"And don't want to have to ride uphill in both directions again." My brain said.

"No I don't." I said to myself shrugging my shoulders. I'd done enough for the day.

When I get home I'm no longer hungry. A glass or two of milk and some raw honey to wipe out the chocolate cravings and I'm good.

My appetite seems to have disappeared.

I feel different too.

Like I have energy for the first time in a while.

Day 5:

14 Miles

1 Hour

Day 6

After closing the restaurant the night before I have to open the restaurant this morning. I had hoped to get up early and ride but reset the alarm thinking that I should try to get at least 8 hours of sleep.

At work all I could think about was the bathroom scale this morning.

205 pounds?

I was up a pound, back to Day 3's weight level and it was wearing on my mind.

Eating small meals a few times throughout the day I still managed to keep my appetite in check.

But would it be enough? I wasn't going to able to squeeze in a ride after work, it would be much too late. Too dark on the unlit bike path next to my house.

Am I going to let this one pound slip ruin my determination?

Or am I going to keep at it?

To be honest, a part of me thought, "Hey, you're off the hook. It didn't work, you tried, but it didn't work."

10 pounds, 10 days.

Maybe it was too much, too fast.

I only had a few more days to go and then the challenge would be over. Why not see it through?

"What else have you seen all the way through?" My brain asked.

It can be a huge ass sometimes, but in a way it was true. I tended to rely on immediate gratification and if the results are too far away from the effort I will usually throw in the towel.

I wanted something to eat, something to drink.

Screw all of this.

But I was stuck at work and it was busy at the bar.

In my anger and self loathing I thought about riding. Being on the bike and riding until sweat oozed from every pore, until every muscle screamed out in agony.

I wasn't going to give up.

Even if I had failed to meet the 10 pounds in 10 days challenge, even if my weight continued to go up, I would still ride.

Because I actually liked it.

And there weren't a lot of things I really liked.

Day 7

To say that relief washed over me would be an understatement.

The bathroom scale read 204 pounds. Not a significant drop in weight but at least it wasn't a gain.

With the rest of the day off I thought I would explore the much longer and never before seen East Bay Bike Path that runs along Narragansett Bay. Starting in Providence it runs to Bristol through East Providence, Barrington and Warren.

The owner of the restaurant had told me it was a brutal 20 miles long in one direction. I was sure he was wrong but he told me had ridden it personally with his son and regretted every minute of it.

The truth is the bike path is 14.5 miles long in one direction and the parking lot at the top of the hill on the Providence side is half a mile up the trail. I didn't think riding the half mile down hill only to turn around and have to ride back up was all that important so I headed towards Bristol with Narragansett Bay on my right.

It wasn't long before I noticed the tingling in my hands. Remembering the two plus hours of numbness from riding the Washington Secondary Bike Path I realized that I was leaning forward, putting too much pressure on my hands.

I didn't want to go through that again and had to concentrate on my posture, and shake blood back into my hands once in a while.

Somewhere in the middle I was glad for the walk signal that seemed to take forever to change. It gave me a chance to rest my butt, even with the padded shorts my cheeks were feeling a little numb themselves. But when the light changed and I started to cross an oncoming Mack truck skidded to a stop, the driver shaking off a yawn that had made him miss the stop light.

Just then the nearby church bells tolled the hour.

"The bell tolls for thee," I thought, "even an off road bike path isn't safe from bad drivers."

The ride was probably one of the most scenic bike paths I had ever been on. At the end there is a diner just off the bike path but of course I had left my wallet back in the car. Maybe that was a good thing, because right now, having completed the 14 miles out to the end I was ready for their largest fish and chips platter with extra tartar sauce.

There are no major hills on the East Bay Bike Path except the one where I parked my car at the beginning. Coming back to that end of the trail I made a silent promise not to get off the bike or let my feet touch the ground.

Already tired and with the hill looming before me I wasn't sure if I was going to be able to make it. So I threw in a little incentive.

"Make it all the way up the hill and back to the car and we'll go out for a ribeye steak."

I could taste it already, juicy, thick and rare.

I tried to gain a little speed before the hill hoping that would carry me up but that momentum was quickly absorbed by the hill. Down shift the gears and keep pedaling.

I don't remember the hill being this long, it seemed to have only taken seconds to ride down it at 26 miles per hour. Now I was climbing it at ever decreasing speeds.

Down shift again and watch the ground slowly move past.

"Not gonna, not gonna." I keep repeating to myself out loud, grunting it. I only caught a glimpse of the lady on the bench just off the side of the trail as I passed her. She must have thought I was nuts.

But I wasn't going to quit, I wasn't going to give up. Not until my speed decreased so much that gravity pulled me over or I was at the top of the hill.

Besides, I wanted that ribeye steak.

Luckily the top of the hill appeared before I fell over and despite the strain I managed to slowly build my speed back up. I felt like I had just won a marathon, I wanted to hold my arms high above my head in victory but knew that I'd probably fall off the bike.

I was feeling a little rubbery.

There was still a little bit of distance until I was back at the car and I noticed for the first time that my body felt different. My thighs were pushing the material on my jeans which a week ago had been baggy in the legs.

Putting the bike back in the car that itchy sensation on my stomach returned, this time up higher as if instead of the bottom of my belly hanging low and rubbing on my jeans or the t-shirt, now it was folding in and rubbing on itself. The itching wasn't so bad as the first time and I almost took it as a sense of accomplishment.

Body fat was leaving.

At the steakhouse I was going to get just a steak, I didn't want a loaded baked potato or mashed potatoes as my side, too many extra calories. I used to get the mushrooms once in a while but only ever ate a few. A salad could be substituted for the potatoes but I usually don't even finish all of the steak if I get a salad.

What the hell I thought, though I wasn't technically hungry I devoured the salad. Eating it was a completely new experience, it was if I was inhaling it. Then the steak came out, 14 oz of ribeye steak cooked rare, looking like far too much. I still didn't 'feel' hungry with the salad in my stomach and thought about taking half the steak home to finish later.

Not a chance, the steak was gone before I could even think about taking some of it home.

What was going on?

Amazed, I realized that though I felt full I could continue to eat unless I kept everything in check. This could be dangerous.

Everyone thinks just because you're fat that you eat tons of food all the time. The truth was I wasn't over weight because I ate a lot, I often had very small portions, the reason was because I didn't do anything physical.

I sat in front of the computer or TV for hour after hour.

There was a story in a magazine about a lady running to lose weight. She had started running and was envious of other runners, how they all had that perfect runners physique and boundless energy. No wonder why they ran all the time.

Then after she had been running for a while and her own body started to change she realized that maybe the reason they had that body and all that energy was because they ran and not the other way around.

Their activity changed their body and increased their energy level.

The hardest part of it all is getting off the couch and forcing yourself to get to that point.

On the way home I picked up a Snickers while getting gas. At home I did the usual, sat my ass down in front of the TV and had a few cocktails.

Things were changing, I could feel it, but sometimes it is tough to let go of the old ways.

Day 7:

28 Miles

2 Hours 14 Minutes

Day 8

Once again I have to open the restaurant, the ten hour shifts were getting in the way of this challenge. Even though I was up early enough to get a quick ride in I decided to take a long shower instead.

Had to recheck the scale a few times to make sure I wasn't imagining it.

200 pounds.

Took a shower and re weighed myself when I got out.

Still couldn't believe it.

I had done it, 10 pounds in... only 8 days.

That's amazing.

But now I'll be stuck behind the bar all day again and wont be able to get to ride. On the positive side all I have to do is manage to hold this weight level, or lose a little more, and this whole 10 pounds in 10 days thing will be a slam dunk.

I was in a great mood all day.

I had done it, my energy levels were up, and while I personally couldn't see any difference in how I looked, I had done it.

10 pounds, 8 days.

Day 9

"Oh no?!"

"It's a mistake." I said and stepped off the bathroom scale.

I stepped back on but the weight was the same, 202 pounds.

Her family had come into the restaurant yesterday and talked about the boat. My confidence level was so high I may as well have set the appointment to go out on the boat in stone.

Now this set back. Was it all really so fragile?

I was in panic mode, and to make matters worse I had to close the restaurant later. If I never had to work this whole thing would be no problem. I'd spend my days riding anywhere I wanted with the best gear and a bike that costs more that $150.

But that was fantasy, this was reality.

What am I going to do now?

Slater Park in Pawtucket had a bike path called the Ten Mile River Greenway. It wasn't a converted rail trail so it had a few hills interspersed along its length. Only once I got there I realized that the name had nothing to do with how long the bike path was, it was the name of the river that ran along its length.

The bike path itself was only two miles long. There was another, unfinished, dirt path extension that was another mile long but sections of it were under water or filled with deep mud. Completely un-ride-able.

But I was there, so...

End to end and back again didn't take 15 minutes.

So I did it again.

A little over half an hour of riding and I had done the whole bike path four times. This was getting boring.

I packed the bike back in the car and checking my watch realized that if I hurried I could get a quick ride in on the Blackstone River Bikeway, out to Martin Street Bridge and back before I had to shower and hustle into work.

I didn't even go inside the house, just took the bike out of the car and headed for the bike path. It was getting late and I didn't like the pressure of feeling rushed. Already people were starting to crowd out onto the bike path, students mostly, just getting out of school, packed in groups taking up most of the path.

Still I was back home within a half an hour.

Not bad but I had hoped to accomplish a little more today.

I just hoped it would be enough.

Day 9:

First Ride

7.5 Miles

30 Minutes

Second Ride

7 Miles

30 Minutes

Day 10

Laying awake in bed I couldn't help but wonder what the scale would say. Sure it was tomorrow that really mattered right? Or was it today?

I weighed in the night before Day 1 at 210 pounds, today was Day 10. Was it today's weight that mattered or tomorrow mornings weight when the cumulative effects of today's exercise would have time to take effect?

I wasn't sure, all I knew was that I should have ridden more, I should have eaten less all week.

Hind sight is 20/20 and all that.

Reluctantly I dragged my ass out of bed and made my way to the bathroom. Never before had I been so intimidated by knowing my weight. Whatever I weighed was just what I weighed.

But now?

Now there was a sort of pressure to have reached a certain goal.

Any other day I could have devoted the entire day off of work to riding some ridiculous amount to try and burn off any last minute calories. Only today I had made plans with an old friend who heard I had started cycling. He wanted to take the commuter rail out of Boston and do some riding around Cohassett, Scituate, and Hull out on the coast of Massachusetts.

It sounded great, originally not realizing that this would be the last day of my challenge, only I didn't know how much cycling we would really do. It could just be a leisurely riding pace that didn't really burn any calories, and on top of that I knew that when him and I got together we usually ate, a lot.

So I stepped on the scale with my eyes closed.

I waited until it had stopped moving, until I was certain that wherever it was pointing at was the final weigh in for the day.

199 pounds.

I laughed out loud and watched the dial shift from my movement.

Deep breathe, let it settle again.

Sure enough it went right back to 199 pounds.

I had really done it. 11 pounds and it was only the morning of Day 10.

Whatever I did today, as long as it wasn't gorging myself on tons of high fat food, would be ok. Whatever the level of riding I would get in would help some, though not as much if I had stayed here and pushed myself to the limits out on the bike path. But friends are important.

Quality of life is important.

I deserve to go out and ride the coast on such a beautiful day and not have to worry about impressing any girl on a boat.

Was that what this was really all about?

Whatever it was I needed it.

Success!

Just getting out and doing it was the hardest part.

Finding the motivation was a big part.

But what really made the 10 pounds in 10 days challenge work was the low blood sugar workouts that increased the amount of calories burned and the "Afterburn" effect of getting the exercise in early and taking advantage of the increased metabolism throughout the day.

Those two leveraged with the high calorie burn of cycling pushed the the limits of how much weight it was possible to lose.

As far as the raw coconut oil goes I can't say, I do know that I didn't do much to curb my calorie intake.

The truth is I was lucky, I had this great off road Blackstone River Bikeway right next door to my house. If more communities invested in the health of their citizens this world would be a much better, and less obese planet.

Saying that it is the communities fault though is just another in the long list of excuses that people find that justify not losing weight now.

Don't have a bike path and are afraid of cycling on the road because of bad drivers? Get a recumbent bike and plant that in front of your TV.

Put in some effort.

Since losing weight a few people have approached me about how cycling hadn't helped them lose weight. To me that just wasn't possible, so I went out with them on a few rides. They were constantly complaining that I was going too fast, getting too far ahead.

They said it was because I had been riding for so long that I was able to go so fast. The truth was they weren't putting in any effort and didn't understand why they weren't seeing any results. I wasn't going fast, keeping the bike speeds at or below 12 mile per hour isn't a lot, even if you are just starting out.

It is speeds of 5 to 8 miles per hour that people seem to think they are riding, really cycling and burning calories.

You're not, you are playing a game with yourself.

14 miles per hour should be your goal for sustained amounts of time.

Not only are you not burning calories if you don't put in the effort you are also not releasing the endorphins that your body craves. Let the exercise become its own addiction.

After a while I couldn't just go end to end and back again on the bike path. I wanted more, and I would go end to end and back all over again clocking 40 miles in a single ride. I wasn't riding everyday like I was during the challenge but I continued to lose weight.

By the end of the summer I was down to 165 pounds.

45 pounds in a little over four months.

That's when I started wondering again about the rest of the East Coast Greenway and my little half joking goal of riding the whole thing.

I was at work wearing a pair of pants that only a month ago would not fit. Previously I had been unable to make the button meet its opposite because I was too fat. Only I was carrying dishes and dropped a cup of water, no problem, I bent over to wipe up the water and my flexing thigh ripped the inner seam of my pant leg from crotch to knee.

Like I was the Incredible Hulk growing out of his clothes.

With my pants split wide open I couldn't help but laugh at how much cycling has changed my physique. Not only had I lost weight but I had gained muscle. How this whole 10 pounds in 10 days challenge had changed my whole life.

The funniest part is that I never did go out on that damn boat.

Never got the girl.

I did however ride my bicycle from Providence, Rhode Island to Key West, Florida to raise money for Meals on Wheels.

But that is another story.

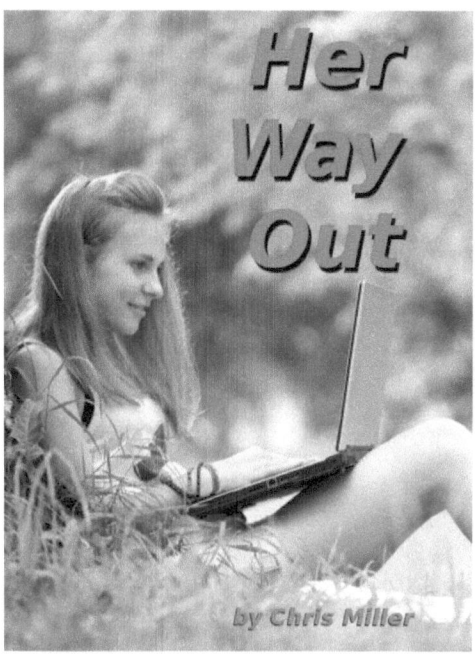

"Suddenly she became aware of her ability to make money online, and as she grew more confident she was able to escape all the little problems that pulled her in too many directions."

That is the sentence that served as the guiding light for the stories that follow, and it is also one that you will be able to confidently say to yourself as you read and apply some of these ideas in your life.

- Have you ever thought about making money online or working from home but found that everyone was trying to "sell" you on their system?

- Have you been swamped by all the options available without knowing which one was for you?

- Have you been unsure about how to get started making money online?

If so these short stories are for you. Each of these five short stories covers a different aspect of how various women started and succeeded in making money online. While each story is fiction they are all based on real life situations that have happened to real women just like you.

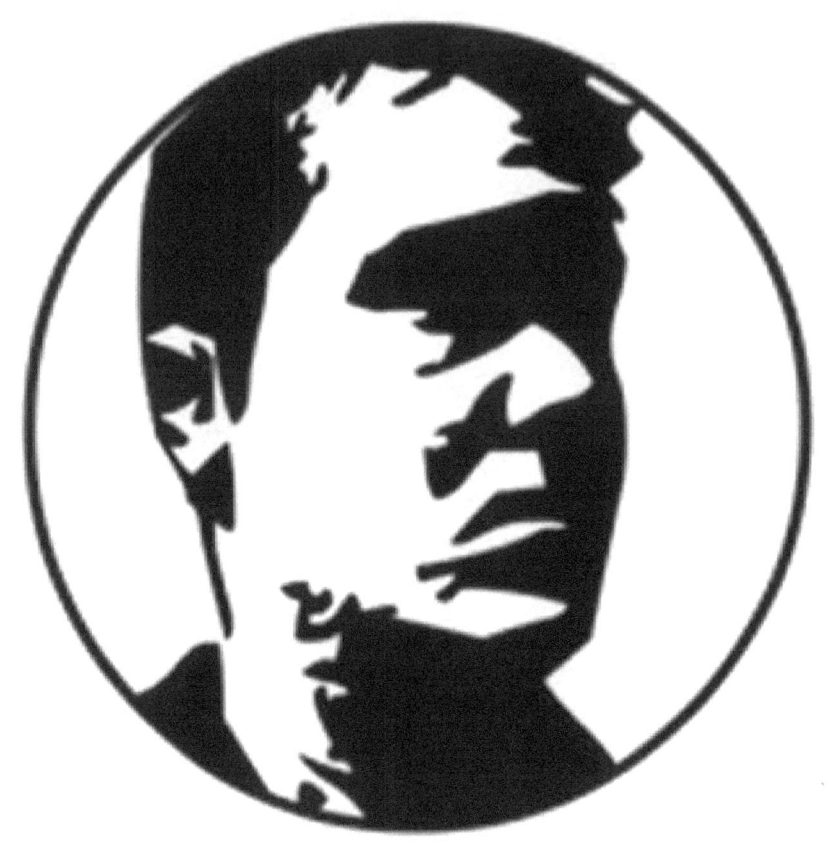

ThingsGoingSmoothly.com